Ana Noelia Hernández González

DUCHENNE MUSCULAR DYSTROPHY:

Ana Noelia Hernández González

DUCHENNE MUSCULAR DYSTROPHY:

From cell to treatment

Imprint

Any brand names and product names mentioned in this book are subject to trademark, brand or patent protection and are trademarks or registered trademarks of their respective holders. The use of brand names, product names, common names, trade names, product descriptions etc. even without a particular marking in this work is in no way to be construed to mean that such names may be regarded as unrestricted in respect of trademark and brand protection legislation and could thus be used by anyone.

Cover image: www.ingimage.com

This book is a translation from the original published under ISBN 978-613-9-41243-3.

Publisher:
Sciencia Scripts
is a trademark of
Dodo Books Indian Ocean Ltd. and OmniScriptum S.R.L publishing group

120 High Road, East Finchley, London, N2 9ED, United Kingdom
Str. Armeneasca 28/1, office 1, Chisinau MD-2012, Republic of Moldova, Europe
Printed at: see last page
ISBN: 978-620-7-98806-8

INDEX

SUMMARY

Duchenne muscular dystrophy (DMD) is an X-linked recessive inherited disease caused by mutations in the gene for dystrophin, a protein essential in stabilising the plasma membrane of muscle fibre during contraction. The disease affects the muscles of the limbs, diaphragm and myocardium, as well as causing spinal deformities and cognitive impairment. Diagnosis is mainly based on clinical suspicion, creatine phosphokinase (CPK) levels, muscle biopsy and genetic testing. MicroRNAs (miRNAs) may be useful in monitoring the disease and therapeutic response. There is no curative treatment for DMD, the gold standard being corticosteroids, which slow disease progression at the expense of possible adverse effects. The design of dystrophic animal models, such as mdx mice, has led to a deeper understanding of the role of dystrophin in muscle and a better understanding of the pathogenesis of the disease. This, together with the lack of a definitive treatment, has increased the interest in designing new therapeutic strategies. The development of gene therapy in recent years has allowed the transfer of dystrophin mini genes contained in adeno-associated viruses, the correction of specific mutations using antisense oligonucleotides or exon skipping techniques, and the overexpression of utrophin. Other therapeutic alternatives include intervention on impaired pathogenic pathways, transplantation with myoblasts or mesoangioblasts, and angiogenesis.

INTRODUCTION

Muscular dystrophies are a group of hereditary diseases characterised by progressive muscle degeneration[1] . Duchenne muscular dystrophy (DMD), the most common muscular dystrophy, is an X-linked genetic disease characterised by a deficiency of a protein located on the cytoplasmic face of the sarcolemma or muscle fibre membrane, dystrophin[1] . The disease affects 1 in 3,500 males and is diagnosed, in most cases, at around five years of age by the observation in the child of delayed motor development, gait abnormalities and a lack of motor skills. inability to run or jump adequately, mainly due to proximal muscle weakness of the lower limbs, as can be confirmed by the classic Gowers manoeuvre. The disease progresses progressively and muscle strength deteriorates to such an extent that children require technical aids for walking and positioning. Later, in adolescence, they require a wheelchair. The average age of death is usually in t h e early twenties, due to cardiorespiratory complications associated with the initial picture[2] .

The overall objective of this review has been to synthesise the current evidence available on DMD. The specific objectives we have set ourselves are: 1) to review the available diagnostic strategies for DMD; 2) to analyse the cellular basis of the disease in order to understand its role in diagnosis and therapy; and 3) to review possible therapies that are currently being developed or tested.

MATERIAL AND METHODS

A systematic review of the existing scientific literature in the Pubmed, Web of Science and Scopus databases was carried out. Search engines such as Google Scholar and Google were also used. The search was carried out in three stages: the first attempted to cover all publications dated from 2000 to 2016 related to the proposed topic. Duchenne muscular dystrophy" was used as the MeSH term; the second search was carried out using the bibliography referred to in the articles of the previous search that were of interest for the present review; finally, the third search was carried out in the same databases discussed above and with the same dating interval, but this time adding the MeSH terms "diagnosis", "therapeutic strategies", "gene therapy" and "stem cell".

RESULTS AND DISCUSSION

1. Results of the search

After the search highlighted in "Material and methods", 62 original articles and 41 reviews were obtained, giving a total of 103 publications. Of these, 65 publications have been used, which are cited throughout this review.

2. Diagnostic strategies at DMD

Diagnosis of DMD is based on clinical suspicion, serum creatine phosphokinase (CPK) levels, electromyography (EMG), computed tomography (CT) or magnetic resonance imaging (MRI), muscle biopsy and genetic study[3] , the latter two leading to definitive diagnosis. The sequence of tests will depend on the technical availability of each centre[4] .

2.1.Muscle enzymes: Creatine phosphokinase (CPK)

Normal serum CPK levels vary with age, sex or physical activity, and may be elevated in various neuromuscular diseases. In DMD, serum CPK is very elevated (50 to 100 times normal values), even from birth[5] . This serum CPK concentration is also seen in other muscular dystrophies present from infancy such as Becker muscular dystrophy (BMD) or limb-girdle muscular dystrophy. However, if there is evidence of proximal muscle weakness in a child, with a "waddling gait", positive Gower's manoeuvre and highly elevated serum CPK levels, we should think first of all of DMD, as it is the most common muscular dystrophy. It is common for CPK levels to fall as the disease progresses due to progressive muscle damage, although values close to normal are only reached in very advanced stages of the disease (Figure 1)[6] .

2.2. Electromyography and imaging techniques

The electromyogram shows a myopathic pattern and is not useful to discriminate the type of myopathy[4] . Imaging techniques, such as CT or MRI (Figure 2), allow us to observe which muscles are affected and to what degree they are affected[3] .

2.3. Biopsy muscle

Muscle biopsy of patients with DMD shows variation in muscle fibre size (some with degeneration or necrosis, and others hypertrophic or with signs of regeneration in an attempt to compensate), infiltration of macrophages and CD4+ T lymphocytes, as well as replacement of muscle tissue by connective or adipose tissue[8] . The earliest alteration found in histological specimens, even before obvious clinical manifestations is the presence of prominent rounded fibres stained intensely with eosin. These fibres contain large amounts of calcium, as demonstrated by Alizarin Red S staining, and their finding heralds the degeneration and necrosis that will occur in later stages of the disease (Figure 3)[6] . In early stages of the disease, there is a balance between the necrotic process of the muscle fibres and the regenerative process. This regeneration will take place from satellite cells that surround the muscle and differentiate into myoblasts to eventually generate small muscle fibres characterised by a central nucleus. Later, the regenerative capacity of the muscle is either exhausted or malfunctions, resulting in new muscle fibres that have an altered contraction/extension complex. As a result, in more advanced stages of the disease, muscle necrosis begins to predominate over regeneration. This is followed by inflammatory infiltration by T-lymphocytes and macrophages, which phagocytose the necrotic fibres, which are eventually replaced by connective and adipose tissue surrounding small islets of non-functional muscle tissue. Thus, pseudo-hypertrophic muscles originate, which at the macroscopic level show excessive weakness for their large size and mass, as seen in the bulky gastrocnemius muscles in some patients [6,7] . The different histological stages of the disease are shown in Figures 4-7. Muscle biopsy can also be subjected to immunohistochemical techniques in order to demonstrate dystrophin deficiency (Figure 8)[4] .

2.4. Genetic diagnosis

If DMD is highly suspected, it is preferable to start with genetic testing, as muscle biopsy is an invasive test[4] . The gene encoding dystrophin is located on the short arm of the X chromosome, in the p21 region, and can undergo various mutations resulting in total or partial loss of the protein, leading to DMD and other milder forms such as BMD[1] .

2.5. MicroRNAs for the follow-up of patients with DMD

MicroRNAs (miRNAs) are small RNA sequences (::22 nucleotides) that act as critical post-transcriptional regulators in processes such as the development, differentiation, proliferation and cell death. Aberrant expression of these miRNAs can be observed in cancer, myocardial infarction and muscular dystrophies. In particular, overexpression of miR-1, miR-133a, miR133b, miR-31 and miR-206 has been found in muscle from patients with DMD compared to control patients. Their importance lies in the fact that they could serve as markers for monitoring and therapeutic response in the disease. The levels of these miRNAs are higher in patients with moderate DMD, whereas, as the disease progresses and complications such as surgical scoliosis or respiratory dysfunction appear, they decrease in response to the loss of muscle mass[12] .

3. Cellular basis of DMD

Clinically and macroscopically, DMD affects the limbs, diaphragm and heart in the form of dilated cardiomyopathy[13] . Muscle weakness can contribute to contractures in neighbouring joints, growth retardation and spinal deformities (e.g. kyphosis)[2] . One third of patients also have cognitive impairment and lower IQ, probably due to mutations in dystrophin expression in the central nervous system. In particular, such disorders are mainly observed in patients with mutations affecting Dp140 and Dp71, isoforms that are abundant in the brain and are structural components of neurons, glia and Schwann cells. GABA-A receptors (y-aminobutyric acid receptors, type A) on Purkinje cells and hippocampal neurons are also decreased. These receptors, through the opening of chloride channels, inhibit nerve impulse transmission, so that their decrease could, in turn, lead to a drop in neuronal excitatory threshold[14] . The cellular bases that could explain the physiopathology of the disease and its corresponding clinical manifestations are detailed below.

3.1.Dystrophin and DAP complex (dystrophin-associated protein complex dystrophin)

During muscle contraction, the contractile machinery of the sarcomere must remain intimately connected to the membrane and extracellular matrix. Otherwise, the movement would be transmitted incorrectly and the muscle cell membrane could be damaged. In this sense, dystrophin is a protein with a component It is a fundamental structural element, since it is responsible for the attachment of the muscle fibre cytoskeleton to the extracellular matrix, stabilising the plasma membrane and thus preventing muscle damage during each contraction. It is also involved in intracellular signalling mechanisms. Actin microfilaments (F-actin) bind to the N-terminal end of dystrophin, while its C-terminal end is bound by the DAP complex, which in turn binds to laminin in the extracellular matrix, specifically the basal lamina surrounding each muscle fibre[15] . The DAP complex includes a number of dystrophin-binding proteins: dystroglycans (a and □), sarcoglycans (a, □, y and ô), biglycan, sarcospan, dystrobrevin, syncoilin, utrophin, Grb2, dysferlin, syntrophins (a, □1, □2, y1, y2) and neuronal 6-oxide-nitric synthetase (nNOS). The sarcoplasmic portion of the DAP complex includes nNOS, syntrophins and dystrobrevin, while the remaining proteins are anchored to the sarcolemma[16] .

On the other hand, the proteins of the DAP complex, together with other additional proteins (vinculin, desmin, etc.), constitute a kind of rib-like latticework (costameres) that extends from the cytoplasmic face of the sarcolemma to the Z-zones of the sarcomere. These costamers also anchor the cytoskeleton to the extracellular matrix and mechanically integrate the contractile action of adjacent myofibrils[8] .

As for 6-oxide nitric synthase (NOS), there are three isoforms: neuronal (nNOS), endothelial (eNOS) and inducible (iNOS). The nNOS and eNOS are constitutive isoforms, whereas iNOS is the only isoform that is expressed in the muscle cell as a result of the inflammatory process seen in the pathophysiology of DMD. The predominant isoform in skeletal muscle fibre is nNOS[17] . It is associated on the one hand with the DAP complex (via a-syntrophin) and on the other hand with caveolin-3. Through a Ca-dependent activity^{2+} /calmodulin, nNOS synthesises nitric oxide (NO) from L-arginine. NO, in turn, is involved in the regulation of glucose metabolism, muscle vascular perfusion during contraction and mitochondrial function. The correct sarcolemmal localisation of nNOS is essential for its proper function[18] .

The last structural component of the plasma membrane is the caveolae, which are nothing more than invaginations of the plasma membrane, consisting mainly of a structural protein (caveolin-3) and cholesterol, sphingolipids and enzymes involved in intracellular signalling such as Src-kinase (tyrosine kinase)[19] . In

DMD, the absence of dystrophin expression and, with it, the loss of functionality of the DAP complex and the disruption of the costamers, would be the basis for the predisposition to plasma membrane fragility at each muscle contraction.[8]

In DMD, the absence of dystrophin expression, and thus the loss of functionality of the DAP complex and the disruption of the costameres, would be the basis for the predisposition to plasma membrane fragility at each muscle contraction.[8]

3.2. Experimental mice for the study of muscular dystrophy

In order to study DMD at an experimental level and to better understand its pathogenesis, the mdx mouse has been designed. This mouse model, resulting from a mutation in ex6n 23 of the dystrophin gene, is the most widely used model for the study of the disease, given its genotypic similarity to humans and the relative ease with which these animals are available in the laboratory. However, its phenotype is milder than that of DMD patients, which could be explained by several reasons: a) mouse muscle satellite cells may have a greater ability to divide and repair damaged fibres; b) the smaller size of mice, compared to humans, means that the forces induced on their muscles are also lower, as is the muscle damage generated. In fact, it is believed that short humans are partially protected against DMD-induced damage; and c) in mdx mice, high levels of utrophin, a protein structurally similar to dystrophin, have been found, so that utrophin-based compensation of the dystrophin deficit may occur. In fact, mice with simultaneous deficiency of both proteins show forms of severe muscular dystrophy that more closely resemble human muscular dystrophy[20].

The relationship between eccentric muscle contraction processes and membrane-generated damage in DMD muscles is a key issue in pathogenesis and has been demonstrated in numerous studies with mdx mice. Immobilisation by injecting toxin into the hind legs of mdx mice has been shown to markedly reduce signs of muscular dystrophy. These studies were performed on mice as young as 3 weeks of age, suggesting that the onset of muscular dystrophy may be due to increased physical activity of the mice after the toxin was injected into the hind legs. weaning. However, this protective effect of immobilisation may also be related to the fact that the fibres immobilised in the mouse are small calibre fibres which, in turn, tend to be less affected by DMD (extraocular, oesophageal striated or distal limb muscle fibres), whereas proximal (large calibre) muscle groups tend to be the main ones affected and have not been taken into account in this study[8] . In patients with DMD, serum CPK levels are elevated immediately after birth, before the physical activity of the child begins. Therefore, a simple dystrophin deficiency would be sufficient to produce the disease without the intervention of an external mechanical force[20] . Even so, inadequate or excessive physical therapy could contribute to the exacerbation of the degenerative process and be detrimental to the patient[2] .

3.3.Increased sarcolemmal permeability as a pathogenic mechanism of the disease

The increase in CPK that occurs in DMD suggests that there must be an increase in permeability in the plasma membrane of the muscle that allows soluble enzymes such as CPK to pass from the cellular interior into the blood. The mechanism by which this increased permeability occurs following contraction has been the subject of much controversy[20] . Over the years, the idea that this increase in permeability could be due to daphnia in the form of pores in the sarcolemma, generated by eccentric contractions on muscles deficient in dystrophin and, therefore, more susceptible to daphnia, has been advocated. At the experimental level, McNeil and Khakee, as early as 1992, demonstrated the increased permeability of the sarcolemma after eccentric contractions in normal muscles, by means of studies in which they observed how substances such as plasma albumin, for which the membrane is usually impermeable, could be found inside the muscle cell. They attributed this increased permeability to the small holes created in the membrane as a result of these contractions[21] .

In order to elucidate whether the holes in the membrane were really the cause of the increased permeability of the membrane, a new study was carried out in which, with the help of a laser, perforations were induced at the level of the sarcolemma, in order to check, by means of fluorescent markers, whether these perforations were repaired and the period of time required to do so. Both in normal muscles and in mdx mice, repair of the holes occurred within a minute. According to the perforation hypothesis advocated by McNeil and Khakee, one would expect that, following eccentric contraction, an extracellular dye would rapidly enter the muscle fibre through the pores, become trapped inside the muscle fibre after repair and maintain constant levels inside the cell. However, the experimental results show a very different dye entry dynamics: immediately after contraction, the dye entry is minimal and then increases progressively without reaching constant levels inside the muscle fibre. Moreover, this dye entry dynamic coincided with an increase in calcium influx into the cell and an increase in reactive oxygen species (ROS)[22] , whereas either blocking stretch-activated calcium channels or using antioxidants largely prevented dye entry into the cell (Figure 10)[20] . The latter theory disproves the hypothesis of stress-induced perforations, and argues for the involvement of calcium and ROS in the increased permeability of the sarcolemma[23,] .[24] .

3.4. Possible sources of increased ROS and intracellular calcium

In the absence of dystrophin, nNOS delocalises from its usual location in the sarcolemma associated with a-syntrophin and caveolin-3 to the sarcoplasm and accumulates there. Its cytoplasmic localisation prevents it from performing its usual functions. Thus, during muscle contraction, the muscle's blood supply is compromised, causing ischaemia. Subsequently, at the onset of muscle relaxation, there will be a sudden reperfusion phenomenon based on oxygen-rich blood. The repeated sequence of ischaemia/reperfusion events will result in the generation of large amounts of ROS that are potentially damaging to the muscle fibre and are involved in increasing sarcolemmal permeability[17].

On the other hand, in DMD, there is an overexpression of caveolin-3. This protein is bound at one end to nNOS and at the other to the WW domain of B-dystroglycan, where it competes with dystrophin. The binding of dystrophin or caveolin-3 to B-dystroglycan is regulated by phosphorylation by srckinase of a tyrosine residue (Y890) in the WW domain. Phosphorylation of this residue will allow the binding of caveolin-3 but not caveolin-3. dystrophin. Therefore, in DMD, a dystrophin deficit and an overexpression of caveolin-3 will coexist[25]. This caveolin-3 overexpression will in turn influence the production of NO by nNOS, the activity of stretch-activated calcium channels and the generation of ROS. Firstly, caveolin-3 has been shown to bind to nNOS and to inhibit nNOS activity. Therefore, overexpression of caveolin-3 would be expected to lead to a decrease in nNOS activity. However, a deficit of dystrophin or asyntrophin is also necessary for nNOS to be affected, since overexpression of caveolin-3 alone does not alter the enzyme[20]. Secondly, virtually all types of transient receptor potentials (especially type 1, TRPC1) - stretch-activated calcium channels - contain a domain capable of binding to src, whose phosphorylation would also overstimulate these channels, allowing calcium to enter the muscle fibre and increasing sarcolemmal permeability[26]. Thirdly and finally, NADPH oxidase, specifically its Nox2 form, is an ROS-producing enzyme whose main activating protein (rac1) is located at the level of the caveolae and bound to caveolin-3. Therefore, overexpression of caveolin-3 will again lead to an increase in ROS[27]. Importantly, ROS generation may also contribute to TRPC1 channel activation, as ROS induce activation of the caveolae src[20]. In addition to ROS and calcium influx as mechanisms favouring sarcolemmal permeability, a calcium-dependent cytosolic phospholipase A2 (cPLA2) is also involved, which, in response to increased intracellular calcium, would use membrane phospholipids to generate lyso-phospholipids and potentially damaging free fatty acids[20] .

In relation to the role of calcium and ROS in DMD, mitochondria, organelles that are essential for energy metabolism and the proper functioning of muscle contraction[28] , are also involved and function as a calcium reservoir, supplying calcium to the cellular interior or removing it from the cytoplasm when necessary[29] . In DMD, the oxidative capacity of mitochondria is impaired as a consequence of excessive intracellular calcium, as observed in mdx mice. Elevated calcium levels are thought to activate mitochondrial transient permeability pores, increasing mitochondrial permeability. and altering its function. This reduces ATP production and leads to an increase in ROS [30,31] .

3.5. Involvement of other channels in intracellular calcium spiking and sarcolemmal permeability

For muscle contraction to take place, the action potential generated at the neuromuscular junction needs to propagate through the sarcolemma into the T-tubules. There, it activates the dihydropyridine receptor (DHPR), a voltage-sensitive L-type calcium channel, whose sensor moves and interacts with the ryanodine receptor (RyR1), promoting its opening and inducing a rapid release of micromolar concentrations of calcium from the sarcoplasmic reticulum (SR) into the cytoplasm. This allows actin and myosin to interact, leading to muscle contraction. Subsequently, calcium reuptake into the SR via the calcium ATPase pump (SERCA) will allow muscle relaxation[32] . Despite the need for strict control of calcium homeostasis during contraction-relaxation processes, small elevations of cytoplasmic calcium in resting muscle may be beneficial in positively regulating thermogenesis, increasing mitochondrial biogenesis or increasing fatigue resistance [33,34] . However, in DMD we find elevated intracellular calcium concentrations that are damaging to muscle[35] . This increase in calcium is initially due to the activation of stretch-activated calcium channels. However, the fact that non-specific blockers reduce intracellular calcium concentrations suggests that other channels may also be indirectly involved, such as the sodium/calcium exchanger and voltage-gated calcium channels. L. In fact, it has been observed that in the cardiac muscle of mdx mice, L-type calcium channels remain activated for a longer period of time than normal, despite the fact that the duration of the action potential is not affected[13]. On the other hand, recent studies from January 2016 reveal a possible link between connexins and the increase of calcium inside the cell. Connexins are non-selective haemichannels permeable to calcium and sodium. In particular, the presence of connexins 39, 43 and 45 has been demonstrated in biopsies from patients with DMD. This is related to an increase in the activation of NF-KB (nuclear factor kappa beta), iNOS and cell apoptosis. In addition to increasing intracellular calcium, these haemichannels may also increase the influx of sodium into the cell, which could lead to an increase in the cellular apoptosis. which, in turn, interferes with the outward removal of calcium normally carried out by the sodium/calcium exchanger. The design of mdx mice deficient in connexins 43 and 45 has reduced the inflammatory activation and oxidative stress characteristic of DMD[36].

In relation to RyR1 receptors, it has been shown that their excessive oxidation or nitrosylation can lead to their over-activation and thus to calcium "leakage" from the SR to the sarcoplasm. Such oxidation arises from alterations in nNOS, caveolin-3, NADPH oxidase and TRPC1, as discussed above[20]. IP3 (inositol 1,4,5-trisphosphate) receptors, located in the sarcoplasmic reticulum membrane, like SERCA or ryanodine receptors, have also been studied. These receptors are activated by IP3, a product of phospholipase C (PLC), and PLC inhibitors have been shown to lead to a reduction in intracellular calcium in the cardiac muscle of mdx mice[37].

Finally, sarcoplasmic reticulum calcium ATPase pump (SERCA1) expression levels appear to be decreased in mdx mice. Therefore, overexpression of SERCA1 may be protective against muscle degeneration (Figure 12)[35] .

Mazala et al. in a 2015 study included three groups of mice: mdx, wild type (no genetic modification), and mdx/Utr mice (with simultaneous utrophin and dystrophin deficiency, whose phenotype more closely resembles that of humans with DMD). Each group of mice was crossed with a strain overexpressing SERCA1, and compared with a control group38. The results of the study are shown in figures 13 and 14.As we can see, much research has been carried out on the role of calcium in DMD, finding multiple mechanisms involved. It is possible that there are still unknown pathways that may be linked to those already detailed in this review[13] .

3.6. Pathophysiological effects triggered within the muscle fibre

The increase in ROS and intracellular calcium generates a continuous challenge in the muscle fibre. In particular, the increase in calcium leads to the activation of calcium-dependent proteases called calpains which, under normal conditions, are activated in the muscle fibre. are regulated by an inhibitor called calpastatin. Calpain inhibition could be a therapeutic alternative in DMD[39] . However, several experimental studies related to this issue have found contradictory results[20] .The increased protease activity leads on the one hand to exacerbation of increased sarcolemmal permeability and increased intracellular Ca2+ and on the other hand to disruption of myofibrils and other cellular structures20 . This necrotic process will trigger an inflammatory response involving macrophages, T lymphocytes and eosin6phils. Depletion of macrophages, CD4+ and CD8+ T cells or any of their perforins reduces histopathological phenomena in mdx mice[40] . In addition, antibody-mediated depletion of T lymphocytes also contributes to the reduction of other inflammatory cells, such as eosin6phils, which promote cell membrane lysis and necrosis. On the other hand, selective regulation of chemokines may also play a key role in limiting the inflammatory response in disease[41] .

Although the specific mechanisms by which inflammatory cells promote dystrophic pathology remain unknown, recent studies support the theory that NF-KB activation, oxidative stress and proinflammatory cytokines (TNF-a, IL-1B and TFG-B, among others) may be mediating this process. Kummer et al., in a 2003 study, found increased activity of NF-KB and other inflammatory cytokines such as TNF-a and IL-1B in necrotic muscle fibres of mdx mice, coexisting with decreased levels of the inhibitory factor IK-Ba[42] . The excessive chronic inflammatory response that occurs in DMD leads to exacerbation of muscle damage, impairment of regeneration and promotion of fibrosis[20] . Fibrosis has a double negative effect on the disease, as it not only impairs muscle function but also reduces the amount of target muscle available for treatments[43] . One of the most important profibrogenic factors in DMD is transforming growth factor beta (TGF-B), which is usually located in a latent state in the extracellular matrix. Conversion to its active form will depend on the muscle damage generated and the activity of inflammatory cells including M2 macrophages. This type of macrophage, distinct from the macrophages classically activated in the inflammatory response (M1), is involved in also in processes such as asthma or pulmonary fibrosis[44] . Activation of M2 macrophages will be provided by cytokines such as IL13, produced by Th2 lymphocytes[43] . Another possible source of activation of these macrophages could be fibrin6gen, as its blockade has been shown to lead to a decrease in TGF-B and thus fibrosis[20] .

Following TGF-B activation, TGF-B can now bind to the TGFB1/2 receptor complex, inducing phosphorylation of the transcription factors Smad2 and 3, and their subsequent binding to Smad4 to be translocated to the fibroblast nucleus and activate the transcription of profibroblast genes[45] .In addition to TGF-B, other factors such as connective tissue growth factor (CTGF) and the renin-angiotensin system are also important players in the fibrotic process in DMD. Angiotensin 2 (Ang2), through its binding to Ang2 type 1/2 (AT 1/2) receptors, contributes to the fibrosis generated in muscle, while angiotensin 1-7 (Ang1-7), an Ang2-derived peptide, inhibits the TGFB-Smad pathway. Thus, the two types of angiotensin have contradictory effects[43] .

3.7. Alteration of muscle regeneration

A fundamental characteristic of healthy skeletal muscle tissue is its ability to regenerate itself in the face of any damage[20] . This is made possible by stem cells called satellite cells, located at the periphery of the muscle fibres and included in the basal lamina. These cells remain quiescent until a challenge is induced in the muscle fibre, at which point they are activated and divide, eventually differentiating into myoblasts. As stem cells, their division is asymmetric, and as they divide they generate differentiated elements (the myoblasts) while maintaining the stem cell pool[46] . The myoblasts, in turn, continue to divide and then fuse to form myotubes, characterised by the expression of different muscle proteins. Eventually, these myotubes will fuse with those of the pre-existing damaged fibres. The fact that several myotubes fuse together explains the central position of the nucleus that is characteristically observed in regenerated muscle fibres. Over time, these nuclei will eventually move to a peripheral position, constituting the typical adult skeletal muscle fibre47 .In muscle biopsies from patients with DMD, regenerated muscle fibres have been observed in very early stages, but as the disease progresses, regenerative phenomena become less frequent. Many studies have been carried out with the aim of clarifying the mechanism by which the regenerative capacity of muscle is depleted in DMD. Blau et al., comparing muscle biopsies from patients with DMD and control patients, found a decrease in the number of myoblasts in patients with DMD, even though the quantification of satellite cells was higher. These increased satellite cells may be in a senescent state that prevents them from proliferating. Later, Webster and Blau extended the earlier study by recording the number of duplications that myoblasts in DMD patients and control patients were able to make. In normal muscle biopsies from patients aged 5 years, myoblasts were capable of 56 duplications, and this capacity dropped to 44 and 22 duplications at 32 and 48 years respectively. In contrast, in patients with DMD, at the age of 2-3 years, the number of duplications was 20-40, rising to 14-16 at 10 years. This suggests that the duplicative capacity decreases in proportion to the number of previous duplications to which the cell has previously been subjected[20] .

In relation to this issue, the role of telomeres in muscle regeneration has been studied, given that each cell division produces its own shortening and this could explain the regenerative failure that occurs in advanced stages of DMD. Indeed, the length of the telomeres in dystrophic cells is shorter compared to normal cells, with a faster rate of shortening. Therefore, dystrophic muscles that have undergone longer dystrophy/regenerative cycles have a lower regenerative window of opportunity[48] . The fact that mdx mice have a milder phenotype than DMD patients could be attributed to the greater length of their telomeres. Sacco et al. designed a mouse model with simultaneous deficiency of dystrophin and telomerase (the enzyme that prolongs telomeres), finding a phenotype characterised by worsening CPK levels, muscle fatigue, histopathological findings and scoliosis, among others, and finding some similarity to the human disease phenotype[49] .

4. Treatment of DMD

Treatment of DMD should be early and multidisciplinary, including the administration of drugs, such as corticosteroids, and appropriate respiratory, cardiac, nutritional and orthopaedic management[4] . Corticosteroids have been shown to delay patients' loss of ambulation, reduce the need for spinal surgery and improve cardiopulmonary function as well as quality of life. Its mechanism of action appears to be related to modulation of apoptosis, inflammation, calcium concentration and myogenesis [50,51] .

Treatment is initiated at 4-6 years, and adjusted according to clinical progression and weight. Weight, height, blood glucose and blood pressure should be monitored, as well as calcium and vitamin D supplementation, vigorous treatment of infections, and annual ophthalmological screening for cataracts[4] . After decades in which corticosteroids have been considered the only therapeutic option in DMD, the situation is changing thanks to the emergence of a wide variety of treatments, some of which have shown promising results[20] .

4.1. Therapies not genetic

This section includes therapies that target key pathogenic pathways altered in DMD.

4.1.1. Drugs related to ROS, Ca^{2+} and NO

As mentioned above, antioxidants have shown great efficacy in mdx mice. Of these, NAC (N-acetyl cysteine) stands out, through the direct elimination of ROS, the reduction of protein disulphide bonds and the increase in the intracellular synthesis of GSH (glutathione, antioxidant)[52] . Another compound with antioxidant properties is epigallocatechin gallate (EGCg), the main antioxidant component of green tea, which has been shown to reduce muscle damage in mdx mice[53] .With regard to drugs that reduce intracellular Ca concentrations^{2+} , in addition to the aforementioned inhibitors of connexins 43 and 45 or the overexpression of SERCA1, the RyR1 receptor stabilisers stand out, which under the name Rycals, reduce the release of calcium from the SR and improve muscle function in mdx mice[20] .

Finally, the NO-CGMP pathway is another potential therapeutic target in DMD. Sildenafil and tadalafil are both inhibitors of phosphodiesterase type 5 and thus prevent the degradation of cGMP, relaxing the smooth muscle of blood vessels and allowing blood to enter the muscle. Through this mechanism of action, these drugs have been shown to be effective in mdx mice. Sildenafil improves diaphragmatic function and reduces inflammation and fibrosis, while tadalafil reduces muscle damage after muscle stimulation during ischaemia [54,55] .

In relation to the NO pathway, a phase I study has also been conducted to assess the safety of the combination of isosorbide dinitrate (a nitric oxide donor) and ibuprofen. Among the results of the study were the absence of pharmacokinetic interactions between the two drugs and the absence of adverse effects. Phase II studies are pending to demonstrate the efficacy of this combination as a treatment for DMD[56] .

4.1.2. Drugs that reduce inflammation and fibrosis

Inflammation and fibrosis are two main pathophysiological processes in DMD. Hence the importance of designing new therapies targeting these processes[20] . The involvement of inflammatory cells, such as macrophages, is necessary to produce effective muscle regeneration after muscle damage. However, a chronic and excessive inflammatory response, as in DMD, is detrimental. The aim of anti-inflammatory drugs in DMD is to maintain the beneficial effects of inflammation without excessive inflammation[20] . Within this group of drugs are TNF-a (tumour necrosis factor alpha) inhibitors, such as Etanercept or

Remicade, used in rheumatoid arthritis[57] . On the other hand, the use of NF-KB blockers, as well as stabilisation of the inhibitory factor IKBa, could be a possible therapeutic alternative to corticosteroids. One example is the administration of a small peptide containing the NEMO domain (the main modulator of NF-KB) known as NBD (NEMO binding domain). However, the peak of NF-KB activation occurs very early in patients with DMD (around 2 years) and decreases over time. progressively with age, suggesting the need to institute this therapy very early in order to achieve maximum benefit[58] .

Fibrosis is the main cause of progressive muscle weakness in patients with DMD, with TGF-B being the main activator of the fibrosis process. Several attempts have been made to find a potent inhibitor of this factor. These include osteopontin inhibitors and halofuginone (HT-100), a natural alkaloid that prevents phosphorylation of Smad3[20] . Other possible alternatives against fibrosis include transgenic CTGF depletion or the design of monoclonal antibodies against CTGF (FG3019), and Ang2 inhibition by Losartan or Ang1-7 treatment[43] .

4.1.3. Protein Replacement Therapies

This therapeutic option consists of the exogenous administration of dystrophin-associated proteins. These include biglycan, which is involved in the transcription and structural regulation of multiple components of the DAP complex, such as nNOS and utrophin. Systemic administration of recombinant human biglycan in mdx mice has resulted in improved muscle function. Another protein, mitsugumin-53 (MG53), which acts by repairing the plasma membrane through the recruitment of intracellular vesicles, has also been shown to reduce sarcolemmal permeability in mdx mice20 .

4.1.4. myostatin inhibitors

Myostatin is a protein that acts as a negative regulator of muscle growth. Therefore, its inhibition could lead to a gain in muscle mass in DMD. The use of myostatin antibodies in mdx mice has improved their dystrophic pathology, although human clinical trials show no improvement in muscle strength and no adverse effects. Despite these discordant results, studies have continued with other myostatin blockers, including follistatin, whose transgenic overexpression in mice quadruples muscle mass compared to control mice. Phase 1/2a trials in BMD patients show the absence of adverse effects, the improvement in the 6-minute walk test and the histological benefits found in muscle biopsies [18,59] .

4.2.   Genetic therapies

4.2.1. Gene replacement with viral vectors

The dystrophin gene is very long (13 kB), which makes its complete restoration difficult. The fact that the partial loss of dystrophin that characterises BMD is accompanied by a milder phenotype has led to the design of mini dystrophin genes which, although lacking many of the spectrin repeats that characterise the protein, allow it to retain some functionality[20] . Direct injection of these mini genes into the affected muscle would only reach the cells close to the site of puncture, requiring several injections[15] . To avoid this, the mini genes would be packaged inside plasmids or viral vectors (lenti and adenoviruses)[20] . Although the results have been satisfactory in mdx mice (increased transgene expression in 65% of fibres and increased muscle resistance to contraction), at the clinical-experimental level the results are somewhat different. In a clinical experiment, 6 patients with DMD were administered a mini dystrophin gene contained in an adenovirus serotype 2. The injection was made into the biceps and, 42 days after administration, a biopsy of the biceps muscle was taken for comparison with the same contralateral, non-intervened muscle. Only in some patients was a mild and transient expression of dystrophin detected, while all developed a strong immune response to the viral vector. The possibility of a life-threatening immune response has precluded systemic administration of lenti and adenovirus as treatment in DMD for the time being[60] .

4.2.2. Stop codon deletion

Fifteen percent of DMD patients have a nonsense mutation characterised by the appearance of a stop codon and the production of a truncated protein with altered function[20] . Initially, it was thought that these patients might benefit from antibiotics such as gentamicin, which is able to continue mRNA reading while ignoring the premature termination codons. However, to achieve such an effect, high doses and chronic maintenance were necessary, which in turn entailed the risk of renal failure and irreversible ototoxicity[61] . To avoid this, ataluren (PCT124), a drug that achieves the same effect, is administered orally and has been well tolerated by healthy volunteers and patients with DMD. Its response is bell-shaped, with the low dose being the most optimal. The Spanish Agency for Medicines Agency (EMA) granted ataluren in August 2014 the licence to become an authorised medicine for DMD [18,62] .

4.2.3. Exon skipping

Most patients with DMD have a deletion-type mutation, so if the exon with the mutation is skipped during mRNA reading, a shortened dystrophin could be obtained, but with some functionality, as in BMD. Drugs such as eteplirsen, an antisense oligonucleotide that prevents the expression of ex6n 51, have shown a slight improvement in the results obtained in the 6-minute walk test. However, although this is the most promising gene therapy in DMD, more studies are still needed to support its efficacy[63] .

4.2.4. Utrophin overexpression

Overexpression of utrophin in mdx mice has shown significant benefits at the muscle level. The first drug developed for this purpose was SMT C1100, which has been shown to be safe and well tolerated. Studies are currently underway to test its efficacy in patients with DMD.[20]

4.3. Transplantation with myoblasts

Myoblast injection has achieved satisfactory results in mdx mice, but not in DMD patients, for several reasons: (a) intramuscular injection of myoblasts triggers a large immune response against the graft, leading to death within 72 hours of most injected cells; b) DMD eventually affects a wide variety of muscles, so a large number of cells would have to be obtained from the donor and placed in each and every one of them; and c) myoblasts cannot pass through blood vessel walls to reach the muscles, so their systemic administration is also ineffective. This makes it impossible to treat DMD by transplantation with myoblasts[51] .

4.4. Transplantation with mesoangioblasts

Mesoangioblasts (MAB), mesenchymal stem cells, are able to pass through the walls of blood vessels and distribute to all muscles of the body from a single administration. To do this, they require the activation of the endothelium. vascular, a fact that occurs in the inflammatory process characteristic of DMD. Intra-arterial injection of MABs has shown satisfactory results in animals with DMD. Recently, an early phase I/II clinical trial has been conducted in Italy, aiming to determine whether MABs from healthy donors are safe as a treatment for DMD. Five patients were included who were given 4 infusions of MABs from HLA-matched donors, following immunosuppression with tacrolimus. Only one patient developed a thalamic infarction after the last infusion. The most frequent cause of cerebral ischaemic events in patients with DMD is atrial fibrillation in the context of cardiac involvement. Stress during the procedure and anaesthesia could have triggered the arrhythmia in this patient. In addition to confirming the safety of administering MAB in humans, the study also introduces a novel intra-arterial route of administration, as until now, administration via the venous route only trapped it in the lung as a first capillary filter and prevented it from reaching the target tissue. Although the clinical trial was not intended to study the efficacy of MABs, indicators of minimal efficacy were observed in younger patients, suggesting that the decreased regenerative capacity and fibrosis that occur in the later stages of the disease may limit the efficacy of this therapy. Furthermore, it is not known whether pre-transplant immunosuppression regimens influence the extravasation of MABs into the target tissue. Therefore, further studies are needed to discuss MAB transplantation as an effective therapy in DMD.[64.]

4.5. Angiogenesis

Studies in mdx mice show a decrease in muscle vascular density and vascular endothelial growth factor (VEGF), which appears to be the result of disease progression over the years. This has increased interest in the design of therapies to increase vascular density at the muscle level65 . VEGF, an essential factor in blood vessel formation, has two types of receptors: VEGFR-1 (Flt-1), which has a proangiogenic effect, and VEGFR-2 (Flk-1), which can act negatively on angiogenesis. Thus, gene transfer of VEGF contained in adeno-associated viruses to mdx mice has been shown to increase the number of blood capillaries, muscle strength and regenerative capacity, as well as a decrease in necrotic areas[65] . Another alternative is the modulation of VEGF receptors. For this purpose, mdx mice and mice heterozygous for the deficiency of Flt-1, the angiogenesis antagonist receptor, have been cross-bred. The mice obtained from the crossbreeding showed an increase in vascular density in their muscles and satellite cells, as well as a decrease in the severity of their phenotype[65] . All these data support the idea that angiogenesis could constitute a therapeutic strategy in DMD, although further studies are needed before these drugs can be applied in humans[65] .

CONCLUSIONS

The following conclusions can be drawn from this work:

1. The absence of dystrophin in DMD patients results in multiple alterations in sarcolemmal properties, intracellular signalling pathways and many other aspects of proper muscle function.

2. Over the years, it has been widely accepted that the first consequences of dystrophin deficiency on muscle fibre are due to the damage generated by eccentric contractions in susceptible muscles. However, although this sequence of events may influence the progression of the disease, more and more researchers support the idea that dystrophin deficiency itself, and the consequent alteration in the regulation of Ca2+ , ROS and NO, are the main causes of the pathophysiological effects that occur in DMD.

3. In addition to clinical suspicion, analytical determination of CPK, muscle biopsy and genetic testing as fundamental constituents in the diagnosis of the disease, microRNAs are emerging as new markers useful for the follow-up and monitoring of the therapeutic response of DMD.

4. The development of gene therapy, increased understanding of the biochemical and molecular implications of dystrophin and interest in stem cell therapies has led to the design of new therapeutic strategies for DMD, some of which have been successful in studies with mdx mice, while others are in clinical trials. After many decades in which corticosteroids have been the only drugs capable of slowing disease progression, optimism is growing among researchers and patients with therapies such as exon skipping, mesoangioblast transplantation or ataluren, already approved as a targeted drug for DMD patients carrying a nonsense mutation. Further studies are probably needed to increase the effectiveness of some of these therapeutic strategies in DMD, as well as the great effort of pharmaceutical companies to prevent their high economic cost from preventing their use by those patients who need them most.

BIBLIOGRAPHICAL REFERENCES

1. Durbeej M, Campbell KP. Muscular dystrophies involving the dystrophin-glycoprotein complex : an overview of current mouse models. Curr Opin Genet Dev. 2002;12(3):349-361.

2. Chaustre DM, Chona WS. Duchenne muscular dystrophy. Perspectives from rehabilitation. Rev Fac Med. 2011;19(1):45-55.

3. Erazo-Torricelli R. Update on muscular dystrophies. Rev Neurol. 2004;39(9):860-871.

4. Rezende JA, Avila BCC de, Alves LB, Silveira FSA. Duchenne muscular dystrophy. An Simpac. 2015;2(1):47-54.

5. Dobrescu MA, Petrescu IO, Tache DE, Farcas S, Puiu M, Stanoiu B, et al. Diagnosis management strategy of Duchenne muscular dystrophy. SRCP. 2015;18(69):9-14.

6. Emery AE, Muntoni F, Quinlivan, RC. Duchenne muscular dystrophy. 4th ed. USA: Oxford University Press; 2015.

7. Vohra RS, Lott D, Mathur S, Senesac C, Deol J, Germain S, et al. Magnetic resonance assessment of hypertrophic and pseudo-hypertrophic changes in lower leg muscles of boys with duchenne muscular dystrophy and their relationship to functional measurements. PLoS One. 2015;10(6):1-17.

8. Deconinck N, Dan B. Pathophysiology of Duchenne muscular dystrophy: current hypotheses. Pediatr Neurol. 2007;36(1):1-7.

9. State University of Campinas [Web site]. Brazil: Department of Anatomia Patol6gica, Faculty of Medical Sciences; 2016 [updated 20 February 2016; accessed 30 March 2016]. Duchenne muscular dystrophy (supporting text); [ca. 4screens]. Available from: http://anatpat.unicamp.br/taduchenne.html

10. Waddell LB, Evesson FJ, North KN, Cooper ST, Clarke TN. Diagnosis of the muscular dystrophies. In: Hedge M, Ankala A, editors. Muscular Dystrophy. InTech; 2012. p. 261-288.

11. Neuromuscular Disease Center [Web site]. USA: University of Washington; 2014 [accessed 23 March 2016]. Dystrophinopathies: Duchenne. [approximately 4 screens]. Available from: http://neuromuscular.wustl.edu/pathol/dmdpath.htm

12. Zaharieva IT, Calissano M, Scoto M, Preston M, Cirak S, Feng L, et al. Dystromirs as serum biomarkers for monitoring the disease severity in Duchenne muscular dystrophy. PLoS One. 2013;8(11): e80263.

13. Van Westering T, Betts C, Wood M. Current understanding of molecular pathology and treatment of cardiomyopathy in Duchenne muscular dystrophy. Molecules. 2015;20(5):8823-8855.

14. Hendriksen RGF, Hoogland G, Schipper S, Hendriksen JGM, Vles JSH, Aalbers MW. A possible role of dystrophin in neuronal excitability: a review of the current literature. Neurosci Biobehav Rev. Elsevier Ltd; 2015;51:255-262.

15. Nowak KJ, Davies KE. Duchenne muscular dystrophy and dystrophin: pathogenesis and opportunities for treatment. EMBO Rep. 2004;5(9):872-876.

16. Kierszenbaum, AL, Tres L. Histology and cell biology: an introduction to pathology. 4th Ed. Canada: Elsevier; 2015.

17. Kim JH, Kwak HB, Thompson LV, Lawler JM. Contribution of oxidative stress to pathology in diaphragm and limb muscles with Duchenne muscular dystrophy. J Muscle Res Cell Motil. 2013;34(1):1-13.

18. Guiraud S, Aartsma-Rus A, Vieira NM, Davies KE, van Ommen G-JB, Kunkel LM. The pathogenesis and therapy of muscular dystrophies. Annu Rev Genomics Hum Genet. 2015;(May):1-28.

19. Gervasio OL, Phillips WD, Cole L, Allen DG. Caveolae respond to cell stretch and contribute to stretch-induced signaling. J Cell Sci. 2011;124(21):3581-3590.

20. Allen D, Whitehead NP, Allen DG, Whitehead NP, Froehner SC. Absence of dystrophin disrupts skeletal muscle signaling: roles of Ca^{2+}, reactive oxygen species, and nitric oxide in the development of muscular dystrophy. Physiol Rev. 2015;96(December):253-305.

21. Allen DG, Whitehead NP. Duchenne muscular dystrophy-what causes the increased membrane permeability in skeletal muscle? Int J Biochem Cell Biol. 2011;43(3):290- 294.

22. Reddy A, Caler EV, Andrews NW. Plasma membrane repair is mediated by Ca^{2+}- regulated exocytosis of lysosomes. Cell. 2001;106(2): 157-169.

23. Whitehead NP, Pham C, Gervasio OL, Allen DG. N-acetylcysteine ameliorates skeletal muscle pathophysiology in mdx mice. J Physiol. 2008;586(7): 2003-2014.

24. Whitehead NP, Streamer M, Lusambili LI, Sachs F, Allen DG. Streptomycin reduces stretch induced membrane permeability in muscles from mdx mice. Neuromuscular Disorders. 2006;16(12): 845-854.

25. Sotgia F, Lee JK, Das K, Bedford M, Petrucci TC, Macioce P, et al. Caveolin-3 directly interacts with the C-terminal tail of beta dystroglycan. Identification of a central WW-like domain within caveolin family members. J Biol Chem. 2000;275(48): 38048- 38058.

26. Gervasio OL, Whitehead NP, Yeung EW, Phillips WD, Allen DG. TRPC1 binds to caveolin-3 and is regulated by Src kinase: role in Duchenne muscular dystrophy. J Cell Sci. 2008;121: 2246-2255.

27. Kawamura S, Miyamoto S, Brown JH. Initiation and transduction of stretch-induced RhoA and Rac1 activation through caveolae: cytoskeletal regulation of

ERK translocation. J Biol Chem 2003;278(33): 31111-31117.

28. Alberts B, Johnson A, Lewis J, Raff M, Roberts K, Walter P. Molecular Biology of the Cell. 5th ed. New York, USA: Garland Science; 2007.

29. Alonso MT, Villalobos C, Chamero P, Alvarez J, Garcia-Sancho J. Calcium microdomains in mitochondria and nucleus. Cell Calcium. 2006;40(5-6): 513-525.

30. Percival JM, Siegel MP, Knowels G, Marcinek DJ. Defects in mitochondrial localization and ATP synthesis in the mdx mouse model of duchenne muscular dystrophy are not alleviated by PDE5 inhibition. Hum. Mol. Genet. 2013;22(1): 153- 167.

31. Bernardi P, di Lisa F. The mitochondrial permeability transition pore: molecular nature and role as a target in cardioprotection. J. Mol. Cell. Cardiol. 2015;78: 100-106.

32. Lanner JT, Georgiou DK, Joshi AD, Hamilton SL. Ryanodine receptors: structure, expression, molecular details, and function in calcium release. Cold Spring Harb Perspect Biol. 2010;2(11): a003996.

33. Bal NC, Maurya SK, Sopariwala DH, Sahoo SK, Gupta SC, Shaikh SA, et al. Sarcolipin is a newly identified regulator of muscle-based thermogenesis in mammals. Nat Med. 2012;18(10): 1575-1579.

34. Bruton JD, Aydin J, Yamada T, Shabalina IG, Ivarsson N, Zhang SJ, et al. Increased fatigue resistance linked to Ca^{2+} -stimulated mitochondrial biogenesis in muscle fibres of cold-acclimated mice. J Physiol. 2010;588: 4275-4288.

35. Cheng AJ, Andersson DC, Lanner JT. Can't live with or without it: Calcium and its role in Duchenne muscular dystrophy-induced muscle weakness. Am J Physiol-Cell Physiol. 2015; 308(9):C699-698.

36. Cea LA, Puebla C, Cisterna BA, Escamilla R, Vargas AA, Frank M, et al. Fast skeletal myofibers of mdx mouse, model of Duchenne muscular dystrophy, express connexin hemichannels that lead to apoptosis. Cell Mol Life Sci. 2016; 1-17.

37. Mijares A, Altamirano F, Kolster J, Adams JA, L6pez JR. Biochemical and biophysical research communicates age-dependent changes in diastolic Ca^{2+} and Na+ concentrations in dystrophic cardiomyopathy: role of Ca^{2+} entry and IP3. Biochem. Biophys. Res. Commun. 2014;452(4): 1054-1059.

38. Mazala DA, Pratt SJ, Chen D, Molkentin JD, Lovering RM, Chin ER. SERCA1 overexpression minimizes skeletal muscle damage in dystrophic mouse models. Am J Physiol Cell Physiol. 2015;308(9): C699-709.

39. Spencer MJ, Mellgren RL. Overexpression of a calpastatin transgene in mdx muscle reduces dystrophic pathology. Hum Mol Genet. 2002;11(21): 2645-2655.

40. Spencer MJ, Tidball JG. Do immune cells promote the pathology of dystrophindeficient myopathies? Neuromuscul Disord. 2001;11(6-7):556-564.

41. Wehling-Henricks M, Sokolow S, Lee JJ, Myung KH, Villalta SA, Tidball JG. Major basic protein-1 promotes fibrosis of dystrophic muscle and attenuates the cellular immune response in muscular dystrophy. Hum Mol Genet. 2008;17(15):2280-2292.

42. Kumar A, Boriek AM. Mechanical stress activates the nuclear factor-kappaB pathway in skeletal muscle fibers: a possible role in Duchenne muscular dystrophy. PHASEB J. 2003;17(3):386-396.

43. Kharraz Y, Guerra J, Pessina P, Serrano AL, Mufioz-Canoves P. Understanding the process of fibrosis in duchenne muscular dystrophy. Biomed Res Int. 2014; 2014:965631. 33.

44. Gordon S, Martinez FO. Alternative activation of macrophages: mechanism and functions. Nature Reviews Immunology. 2010; 32(5):593-604.

45. Leask A, Abraham DJ. TGF-beta signaling and the fibrotic response. PHASEB J. 2004;18(7): 816-827.

46. Skuk D. Myogenic cell transplantation: regenerative medicine in skeletal and cardiac muscle pathologies. Rev Med Urug. 2009;25:181-197.

47. Chan S, Head SI. The role of branched fibres in the pathogenesis of Duchenne muscular dystrophy. Exp Physiol. 2011;96(6): 564-571.

48. Decary S, Hamida CB, Mouly V, Barbet JP, Hentati F, Butler-Browne GS. Shorter telomeres in dystrophic muscle consistent with extensive regeneration in young children. Neuromuscul Disord. 2000;10(2): 113-120.

49. Sacco A, Mourkioti F, Tran R, Choi J, Llewellyn M, Kraft P, et al. Short telomeres and stem cell exhaustion model duchenne muscular dystrophy in mdx/mTR mice. Cell. 2010;143(7):1059-1071.

50. Shapiro F, Zurakowski D, Bui T, Darras BT. Progression of spinal deformity in wheelchair-dependent patients with Duchenne muscular dystrophy who are not treated with steroids: coronal plane (scoliosis) and sagittal plane (kyphosis, lordosis) deformity. Bone Joint J. 2014;96-B(1): 100-105.

51. Sienkiewicz D, Kulak W, Okurowska-Zawada B, Paszko-Patej G, Kawnik K. Duchenne muscular dystrophy: current cell therapies. Ther Adv Neurol Disord. 2015;8(4):166-177.

52. Samuni Y, Goldstein S, Dean OM, Berk M. The chemistry and biological activities of N-acetylcysteine. Biochim Biophys Acta. 2013;1830(8): 4117-4129.

53. Nakae Y, Dorchies OM, Stoward PJ, Zimmermann BF, Ritter C, Ruegg UT. Quantitative evaluation of the beneficial effects in the mdx mouse of epigallocatechin gallate, an antioxidant polyphenol from green tea. Histochem

Cell Biol. 2012;137(6): 811-827.

54. Asai A, Sahani N, Kaneki M, Ouchi Y, Martyn JA, Yasuhara SE. Primary role of functional ischemia, quantitative evidence for the two-hit mechanism, and phosphodiesterase-5 inhibitor therapy in mouse muscular dystrophy. PLoS One. 2007;2(8): e806.

55. Percival JM, Whitehead NP, Adams ME, Adamo CM, Beavo JA, Froehner SC. Sildenafil reduces respiratory muscle weakness and fibrosis in the mdx mouse model of Duchenne muscular dystrophy. J Pathol. 2012;228(1): 77-87.

56. Cossu MV, Cattaneo D, Fucile S, Pellegrino P, Baldelli S, Cozzi V. Combined isosorbide dinitrate and ibuprofen as a novel therapy for muscular dystrophies : evidence from Phase I studies in healthy volunteers. 2014;8: 411-419.

57. Ermolova NV, Martinez L, Vetrone SA, Jordan MC, Roos KP, Sweeney HL, et al. Long-term administration of the TNF blocking drug Remicade (cV1q) to mdx mice reduces skeletal and cardiac muscle fibrosis, but negatively impacts cardiac function. Neuromuscul Disord. 2014;24(7): 583-595.

58. Reay DP, Yang M, Watchko JF, Daood M, O'Day TL, Rehman KK, et al. Systemic delivery of NEMO binding domain/IKKgamma inhibitory peptide to young mdx mice improves dystrophic skeletal muscle histopathology. Neurobiol Dis. 2011;43(3): 598- 608.

59. Mendell JR, Sahenk Z, Malik V, Gomez AM, Flanigan KM, Lowes LP, et al. A phase 1/2a follistatin gene therapy trial for Becker muscular dystrophy. Mol. Ther. 2015; 23(1):192-201.

60. Mendell JR, Campbell K, Rodino-Klapac L, Sahenk Z, Shilling C, Lewis S, et al. Dystrophin immunity in Duchenne's muscular dystrophy. N Engl J Med. 2010;363(15): 1429-1437.

61. Malik V, Rodino-Klapac LR, Viollet L,Wall C, King W, Al-Dahhak R, Lewis S, et al. Gentamicin-induced readthrough of stop codons in Duchenne muscular dystrophy. Ann. Neurol. 2010; 67(6):771-780.

62. Finkel RS, Flanigan KM, Wong B, Bonnemann C, Sampson J, Sweeney HL, et al. Phase 2a study of ataluren-mediated dystrophin production in patients with nonsense Duchenne muscular dystrophy mutation. PLoS One. 2013;8(12):e81302.

63. Mendell JR, Rodino-Klapac LR, Sahenk Z, Roush K, Bird L, Lowes LP, et al. Eteplirsen for the treatment of Duchenne muscular dystrophy. Ann Neurol. 2013;74(5): 637-647.

64. Cossu G, Previtali SC, Napolitano S, Cicalese MP, Tedesco FS, Nicastro F, et al. Intra-arterial transplantation of HLA-matched donor mesoangioblasts in Duchenne muscular dystrophy. 2015;7(12):1513-1528.

65. Shimizu-Motohashi Y, Asakura A. Angiogenesis as a novel therapeutic strategy for Duchenne muscular dystrophy through decreased ischemia and increased satellite cells. Front Physiol. 2014;5 FEB(February):1-7.

ANNEXES

IMAGES AND FIGURES

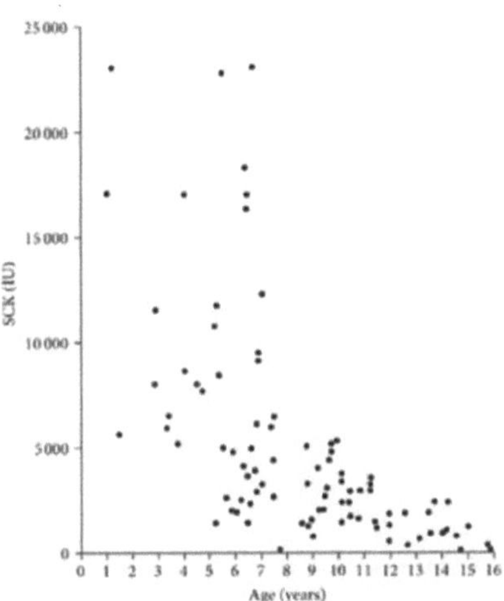

Figure 1. Serum CPK levels in children with DMD. It can be seen how levels decrease as the disease progresses[6].

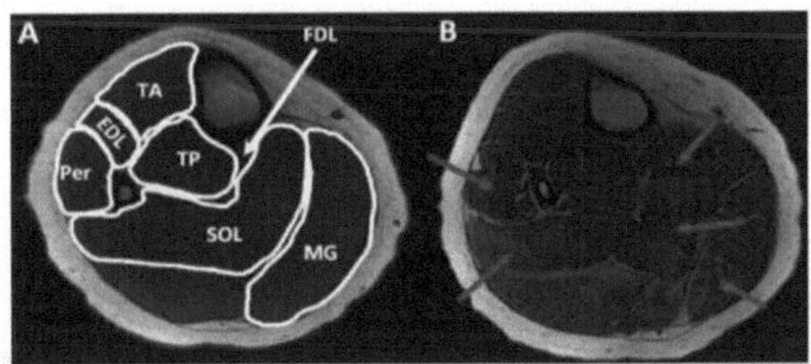

Figure 2. T1 MRI of lower extremity muscles. A) Control patient, and B) Patient with DMD. TA (tibialis anterior); EDL (extensor digitorum longus); Per (peroneus); MG (medial gastrocnemius), SOL (soleus); TP (tibialis posterior); FDL (flexor digitorum longus). In image B, areas of fatty infiltration can be seen at muscle level[7].

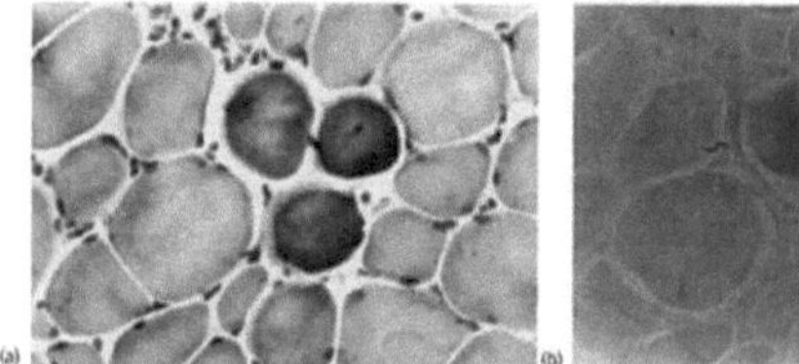

Figure 3. Histological muscle section of a patient with preclinical stage DMD: (a) staining with haematoxylin-eosin; (b) staining with alizarin red S[6] .

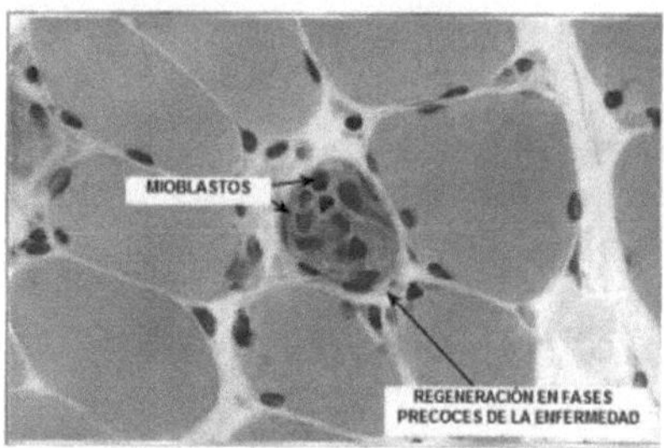

Figure 4. Early stage DMD, H-E staining: an attempt at muscle regeneration from myoblasts is observed[9] .

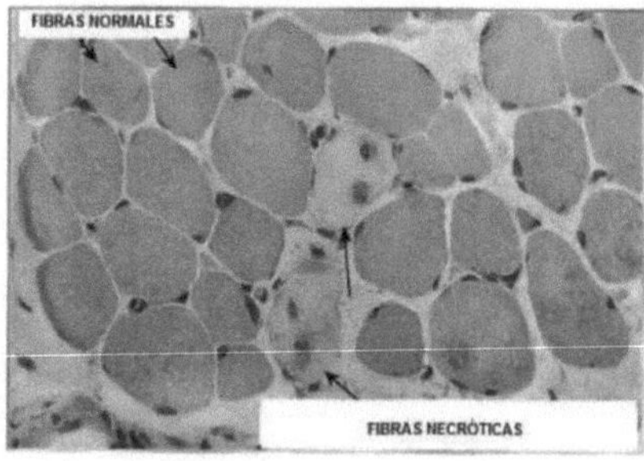

Figure 5. Muscle biopsy of a patient with DMD, stained with H-E: necrosis of some muscle fibres is observed, compared to completely normal fibres[9] .

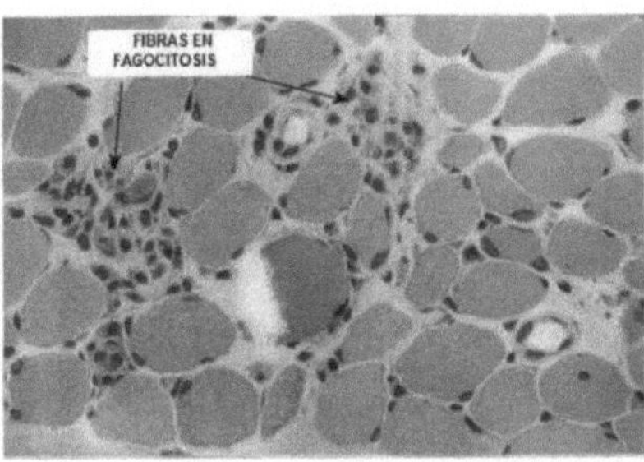

Figure 6. Histological muscle section of a patient with DMD, stained with H-E: macrophages are observed inside necrotic muscle fibres[9] .

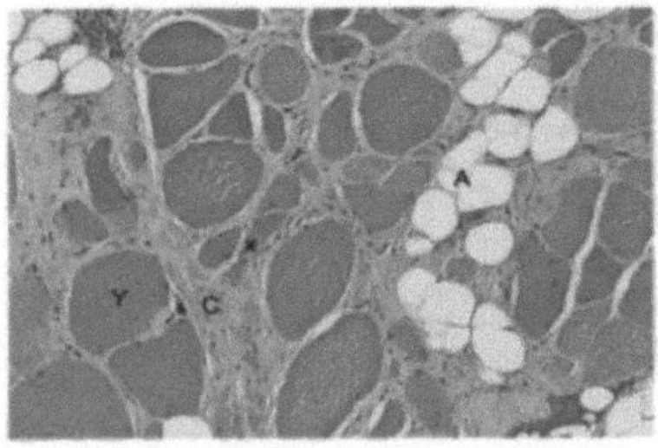

Figure 7. Histological muscle section of patient with DMD, stained with H-E: variation in muscle fibre size, with some atrophic (X) and some hypertrophic (Y), connective tissue (C) and adipose tissue (A)[10] .

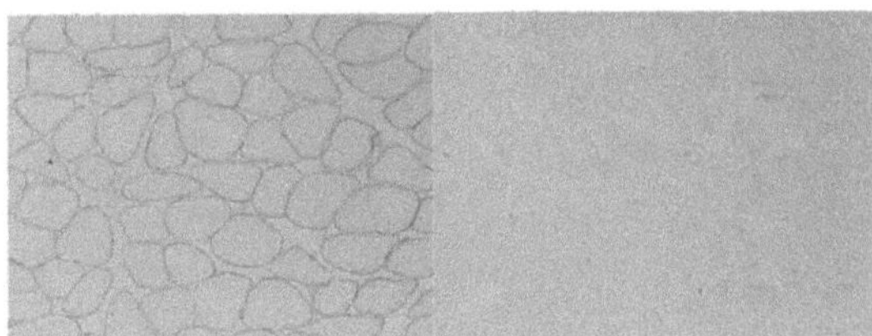

Figure 8. Immunohistochemical test. Left: presence of dystrophin on the surface of muscle fibres, in healthy patient. Right: absence of dystrophin in DMD[11] .

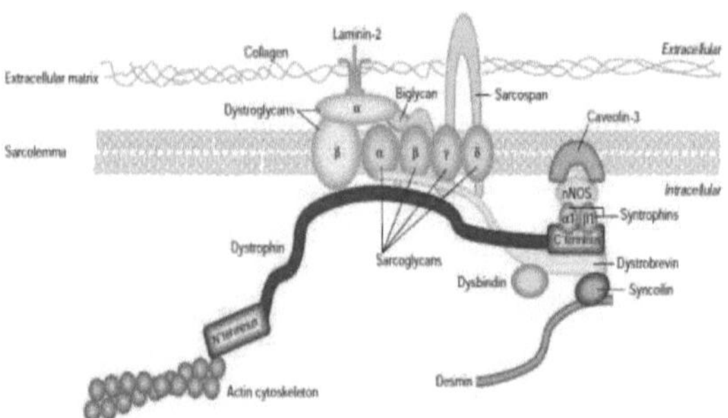

Figure 9. Dystrophin and its relationship to other muscle fibre proteins[15] .

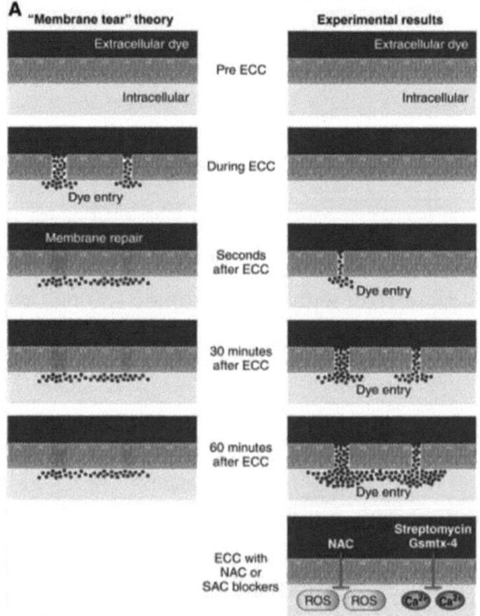

Figure 10. Stretch-induced mechanisms of increased sarcolemmal permeability. Left: according to the perforin hypothesis; right: experimental results. Streptomycin and Gamtx-4 are both stretch-activated calcium. NAC (N-acetyl cysteine) is an antioxidant against ROS20 .

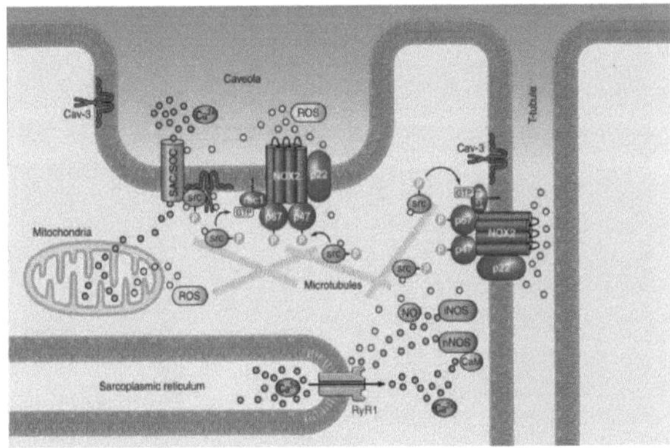

Figure 11. Role of caveolin-3 and nNOS in the increase of intracellular Ca^{2+} and ROS[20] .

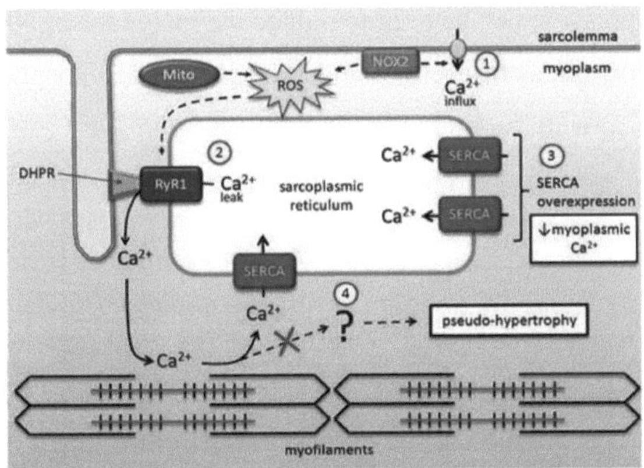

Figure 12. Model explaining the increase of calcium in the sarcoplasm[35] .

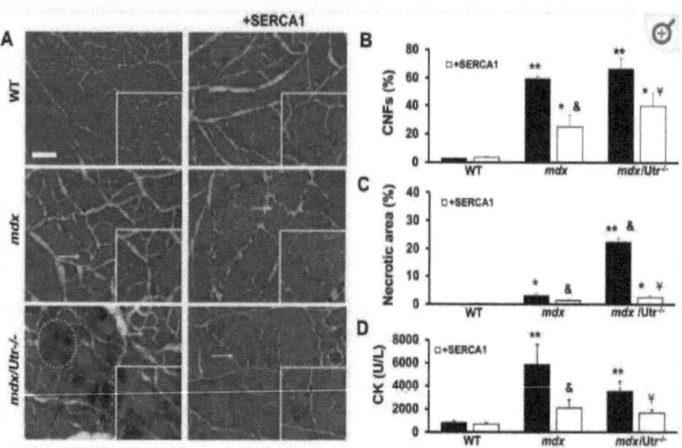

Figure 13. A) Overexpression of SERCA1 in mice with simultaneous dystrophin and utrophin deficiency protects muscle from eccentric contraction-induced damage and reduces areas of necrosis. B, C and D) SERCA1 overexpression can be seen to reduce the incidence of NPCs, pseudohypertrophy, areas of necrosis and plasma creatine phosphokinase levels as well as other markers of muscle damage[38] .

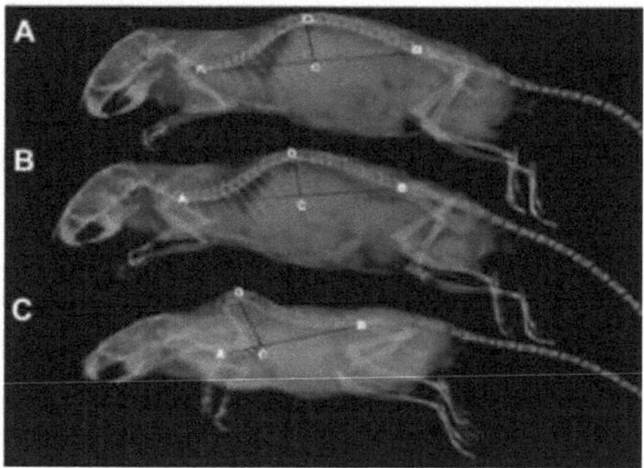

Figure 14. X-rays showing spinal curvature in wild type mice (A), mdx/Utr+SERCA1 mice (B) and mdx/Utr mice without SERCA1 (C). A reduction in kyphosis is observed in SERCA1-overexpressing mice.[38].

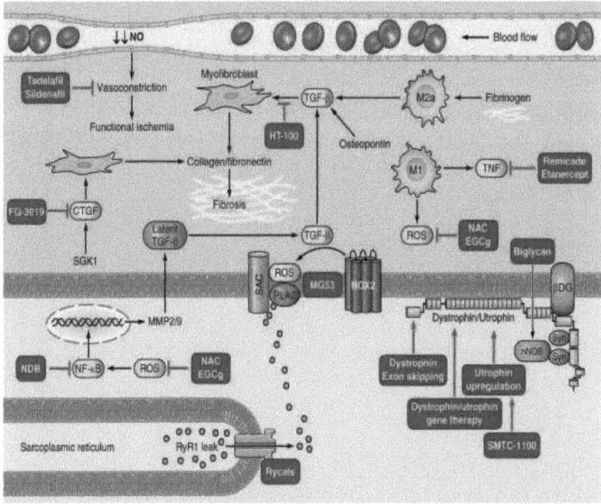

Figure 15. Possible therapeutic strategies for DMD[20] .

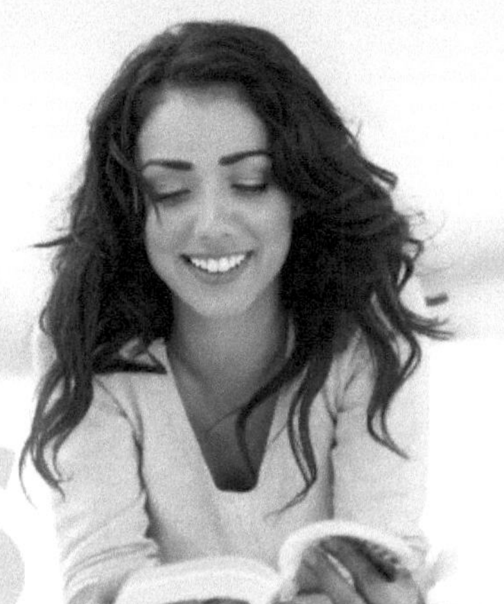

yes I want morebooks!

Buy your books fast and straightforward online - at one of world's fastest growing online book stores! Environmentally sound due to Print-on-Demand technologies.

Buy your books online at
www.morebooks.shop

Kaufen Sie Ihre Bücher schnell und unkompliziert online – auf einer der am schnellsten wachsenden Buchhandelsplattformen weltweit! Dank Print-On-Demand umwelt- und ressourcenschonend produziert.

Bücher schneller online kaufen
www.morebooks.shop

info@omniscriptum.com
www.omniscriptum.com

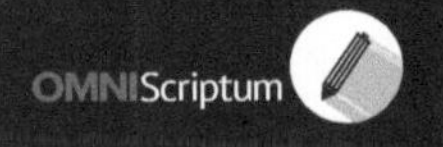

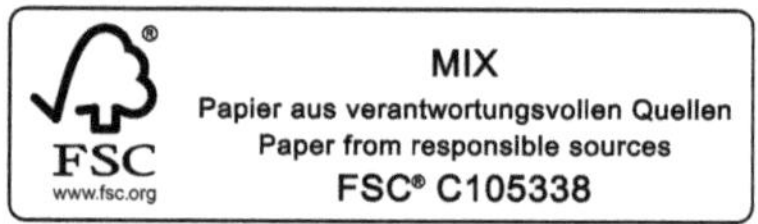

Printed by Books on Demand GmbH, Norderstedt / Germany